THE 9 DAY VIBRANT ENERGY CLEANSE

9 days to lose weight, obliterate <u>anything</u> that's ailing you, and multiply your energy exponentially!

By Andrew Blakehall
Health Coach, Personal Trainer, and developer of the Vibrant Energy Cleanse

The 9 Day Vibrant Energy Cleanse is *vital* for anyone who wants to lose weight, feel amazing, reboot their system, and reclaim their health. Unlike other cleanses, the 9 Day Vibrant Energy Cleanse features helpful videos for every step of the journey. This cleanse is not just a diet, it's the result from years of trial and error in my own life, and in my pro-bono work with clients. Over my decade of experience, I have amassed dozens of tips to make your transition into Vibrant Energy and amazing health as seamless as possible.

Published by Iditatran Press (USA) 948 Hudson Street, New York, NY 10014, Iditatran
Press (Australia) Iditatran Press 19489 Wollumburah St. Sydney NSW, Australia,
(Canada) edition Iditatran, 2010, 39 Rue De Filbraet, Montreal, Quebec, Canada, M4P 24,
(England) 39 Brighton, F2CR OLA

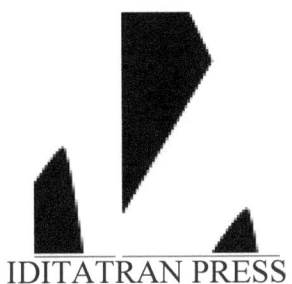

IDITATRAN PRESS

Table of Contents

INTRODUCTION

The 9-day Vibrant Energy Cleanse is an optimized nutrition plan directed to help you achieve your optimum weight, feel as energized as a kid on Christmas morning, and feel healthier than you have years. These aren't mere claims, they are based on my years working with clients who were both overweight <u>and</u> suffering from every malady imaginable. We start by clearing your body of acids lodged in your bones and joints (acidosis). The objective of the second phase is to flush your system of toxins such as candida and parasites, using carefully selected anti-inflammatory herbs. Finally, in the last stage, we replenish your guts flora with a host of healthy macrobiotics.

By Day 9 you can expect to experience:

- A decrease in adipose tissue (fat)
- More energy than you've had in years
- More mental clarity
- Dissipation in all forms of arthritic pain and gout
- Increased libido
- An easier time falling and staying asleep
- Better digestion
- Regulated bowel movements
- Regulated blood sugar
- Measurable absolution of acne, psoriasis, and eczema
- A stronger short-term memory
- Atherosclerosis
- Diabetes (Check with doctor before beginning any cleanse)
- Yeast and\or fungal infections
- Erectile Dysfunction
- Crones Disease
- Osteoporosis
- A stronger buffer against many common contagious diseases such as strep throat, influenza, and the common cold.

3 Reasons Why Traditional Diets Don't Work Long Term

I feel that the traditional diet model is so embedded in the psyches of most dieter's that it would be worth a few paragraphs to shed some light on why it is such a frustrating model. If you have ever participated in a diet in which the goal was to lose weight by cutting calories, and if, after failing, you became skeptical of all diets, cleanses, and fasts, then I invite you to read the section below, so you can understand why 91% of dieters fail at traditional diets.

I have never met a person who has succeeded *long term* in losing a large amount of fat by cutting calories or restricting certain food groups. After years of research I discovered that there are three main reasons why traditional 'Calorie Cutting' diets don't work.

First Challenge: it requires willpower to refrain from eating glucose, however, in order to have willpower, one must consume glucose. This Catch-22 makes perpetual starvation impossible.
My Solution: In this cleanse you will be consuming a lot of glucose. The sugars may be different than ones you are accustomed to. Unlike diets, you will not feel hungry during this cleanse. If you feel hungry you will be advised to eat.

Second Challenge: There is a part of the brain called the *Hypothalamus* that regulates metabolism and fat storage. When the Hypothalamus senses that it is going to be receiving less calories it adapts to the loss by storing fat! Ironically, the bodies gets better at storing fat over time, thereby making it increasingly harder to lose weight over the span of the diet.
My Solution: because you won't be starving yourself, or depriving yourself of base food groups (fats, carbohydrates, proteins) your hypothalamus won't go haywire.

Third Challenge: Most calorie cutting diets do not emphasize nutrition, digestion, or acid alkaline balance. Neither a malnourished body, nor an acidic body can be healthy in the long term, and therefore the dieter is driven to consume foods to try and solve a problem they don't consciously know that they have: Malnutrition.

My Solution: The deceptively simple answer is that we need to stop focusing on cutting out foods and start focusing on replacement.

More specifically, we need to:

1a. Replace 'bad' carbohydrates with high quality, nutrient dense carbohydrates.

1b. Replace 'bad' fats with high quality, omega rich fats.

1c. Replace 'bad' sugars with high quality, non-taxing sugars.

My Background

How Searching For A Cure For My Arthritis Turned Into the format for the 9-Day Vibrant Energy Cleanse

I want to make this book about *you*. I want to help you become *empowered* with the right knowledge so that you can begin a proactive path towards improving your health. However, before I do that, I felt that it would be pertinent to dedicate a few paragraphs to how I came to make some distinctions about diet, health, and inflammation. If you are not interested in about my backstory I invite you to skip forward to page nine.

My journey began on May 9th 1997. I was DJing an 80's night at a `Honolulu nightclub. I was in the middle of a great set and the room was filling steadily. Despite being six feet tall, I couldn't see the entire dance floor. So I hastily decided to stand up on a chair that was a fixture in the DJ booth. Halfway through the song 'Heart of Glass' an assailant entered the booth, reached up around my neck and pulled me down onto the hardwood floor (It was a case of mistaken identity, not a case of disliking my musical selection). My left leg buckled under the weight of my body, and I could feel my bones breaking. The assailant was pulled off of me and held by security, while I was carried down to an ambulance. At the hospital, X-rays showed that I had suffered two hairline fractures in my tibia, and a compound fracture in my fibula. The three breaks were so severe that my doctor claimed that they were 'The worst non-vehicular related bone fractures' he had seen in his twenty-year practice. A titanium rod was inserted into my leg and affixed to the bone with metal screws.

After six months of recuperation, I returned for a surgical bone graft on my fibula to help the separated fragments heal.

Fast forward to January 1999. My prognosis looked great: I could walk without limping, my bones had recovered their strength, my joints weren't grinding or clicking, and my mobility was at 98 percent. In addition to all this positive news, I hadn't experienced any ill side effects. I was twenty-one years old.

In 1999 I relocated from Honolulu to Seattle. About four years after the move, the pain began. At first, it was a numb, almost dull sensation in my ankle and inner knee. Over the course of the following months the pain became more acute. An orthopedic specialist diagnosed me with arthritis. She then went on to prescribe me Vicodin and Ibuprofen. The painkillers helped, but the doctor warned me I couldn't take them forever. The Ibuprofen provided minimal relief at best. I began to look into other options: stretching, heat rubs, Epson soaks, ice packs, massages, etc. I was troubled by the inconsistency of the results. I found that almost all of the treatments alleviated *some* of the pain *some* of them time, but that none of the treatments *solved* the problem. A metaphor I like to use today is placing Band-Aids over an infected wound. Up until that point, all the prescriptions had really just covered the metaphorical infection; none of them had *healed* the wound itself.

My lack of mobility caused me to start gaining weight. Seeing that I was gaining weight, and feeling powerless to do anything about it made me depressed. In my depression, I developed a habit of drinking soda and eating sugary sweets to raise my spirits. This turned into a vicious cycle. I would eat because I was depressed and immobile. This would make me more immobile and more inactive, which would make me more depressed, and would make me want to eat more.

I began searching the Internet for solutions. I made the mistake of entering chat rooms with handles such as *Rheumatoid Suffers Anonymous*. The consensus in these chat rooms was that arthritis (and the resulting weight gain) is an ailment that sufferers must deal with. For a while I succumbed to the spell of the community. When my knee flared up I would swallow my Ibuprofen and rest in (relative) peace knowing that I had done all that I could do. My new goal (if it could be called a goal) was to treat the problem, not to find ways to cure it. The early interactions with my doctor, and the apathetic people in the chat rooms led me to what I like to refer to as my *early viewpoint toward arthritis and my weight gain:*

I had an injury. Because I had an injury, I have arthritis and am overweight. Because arthritis is a permanent ailment, my weight is a permanent result of my condition. I am helpless to change my circumstances.

Come the winter of 2006, I was thirty-seven pounds overweight and the pain was intensifying. On some nights my bones would throb beneath the skin. Sometimes they would fall into a steady, creeping ache. I hit bottom at 3:00 am on December 26th, 2006. The pain actually threw me out of a deep slumber. I flipped on the light and ingested my Ibuprofen and tried to go back to sleep. An hour passed and the pain intensified. I took more Ibuprofen. Thirty more minutes passed and the pain reached a level I never experienced before. I finally sat up and yelled:

"ENOUGH! THERE HAS TO BE SOMETHING I CAN DO! I DON'T CARE WHAT IT IS! I WILL FIND IT!"

I had made a resolution that I <u>wasn't</u> going to settle anymore.

About three weeks later I joined a gym. I had heard that soaking in the Jacuzzi might be therapeutic. On my first day there, a man with a runner's physique came and joined me and some other people in the bubbling water. I'm not in the practice of checking out men in Jacuzzis, but something about this individual intrigued me. He was in stunning shape. (I remember comparing him to Lance Armstrong, which seems ironic now.) I searched the bubbles and wondered if this athlete knew what it was like to live in near constant pain. I felt envious of him. Here he was running marathons while I was in a sort of hell. But when he climbed out of the Jacuzzi to refill his water bottle, I noticed a series of tell tale scars down his right leg. I also noticed a vertical scar on his right knee.

After introducing myself, I learned that he had fallen off a motorcycle at about the same time I had sustained my own injury. Like me, he had broken both his tibia and fibula. In addition, he also had a titanium rod fastened to his fibula to hold it together! After he finished his story I shared my own. I then asked a question which was about to change everything:

"Doesn't running give you really bad arthritis?"

"I don't have arthritis… I mean not *anymore*."

It's been almost a decade and I can still hear him saying that sentence like it was yesterday. My paradigm had been *shattered*. I realized I had been doing it all wrong! Instead of looking for people who *suffered* from arthritis and were overweight, I decided to seek out individuals who had either cured it altogether, or who were proactively curing it. I decided to study three populations:

1. Individuals who <u>had</u> been severely injured, developed arthritis or gained weight, and cured themselves. (What did they do to cure their arthritis or lose the weight?)

2. Individuals who <u>had</u> been injured, yet <u>never</u> developed arthritis or gained weight. (What in their lifestyle prevented these conditions in the first place?)

3. Individuals who had never been injured, yet developed arthritis or gained weight, and then cured themselves. (What were they doing that caused them to develop the disease (or gain the weight), what did they later do to solve the problem.

I knew that if I could find the correlations I could find the answer. I should mention that *I firmly refused to believe that my own arthritis and weight gain was simply the result of injury or my genetics.*

Based on what I learned and observed, I developed a set of principals and began adhering to them. Within weeks I was experiencing results. I modified the results based on what was working and what wasn't. Within 6 months I was arthritis free and back in shape. It has been ten years, and in that time I have run multiple marathons, biked, and hiked, all without experiencing any of the pains that once plagued me. More importantly, the changes I made in my lifestyle didn't just improve my health challenges; I firmly believe that they improved every facet of my health and well being.

Over the years I began posting ads on Craigslist inviting people to try what I am now inviting you to do. I took their feedback, took what worked, threw out what didn't, and really lasered in on making this the most affective health and weight loss program I could. What follows are my results.

Stage 1: Alkaline Stage
(Days 1-3)
Overview

During the first stage, you'll be drinking a lot of purified water, *lemon water*, *green drinks*, and fresh vegetable juice. In addition, you'll be cutting back on coffee and sweetened beverages, reducing processed foods, and eliminating dairy products. You'll be replacing them with *Alkalizing Foods* (Described and listed in Chapter 1)

Benefits you will start to feel by the end of day 3: Increased energy, Increased mental acuity, heightened libido, heightened stamina, relief from caffeine and sugar addiction, relief from adrenal fatigue, clearing candida, stabilizing thyroid issues, replenishing depleted nutrients, and relieving acidosis.

Why Acid Alkaline Balance is important

If you measured your temperature, and the thermometer read 102.5 degrees, my guess is that you would take action *immediately*. You might call for an ambulance. You might put a cold cloth on your head and drink some cold water. You certainly wouldn't ignore it. In our society we accept that a person's body temperature is a good metric for determining the general well being of their vital functions. But there is one metric that I believe to be of equal importance: It is the measure of the Acid\Alkaline balance of the blood. Your body is an electrical power station. Everything is able to move because of a series of biochemical reactions. All the nerves and pulsations happen, in part, because of an electrical balance. The simplest way to describe that balance would be to think of your body as a battery: A battery as you probably know, has two poles: A negative pole, and a positive pole. If you remove some of the charge of either pole, the battery begins to lose its energy.

All of your major organs function because of the electrical charge created by an acid alkaline balance. Each organ and system requires its own unique degree of acidity and alkalinity in order to function. Your blood also has an acid alkaline balance. If that balance is compromised your health is in deep trouble.

The Blood

Your blood serves many purposes, but its primary function is to carry oxygen to your vital systems and to transport waste and\or carbon dioxide away from those systems. Remember how I related your body to a battery? Each of your individual red blood cells is also like a tiny battery. Each cell has an outer, negative charge (Acid) and an inner, positive charge (Alkaline). Because all of your red blood cells have an outer charge that is negative, this permits them to 'push off' from one another. However, because our lifestyles are *extremely* acid forming, our blood cells loose their charge over time, causing them to clump together.

How this pertains to your health

Human blood is slightly alkaline in nature. Some organs, such as the stomach, need to be acidic in order to function properly, but the blood must retain an acid alkaline balance at all costs. If the blood became too acidic, red blood cells would no longer be able to transport oxygen, and everything would shut down. As humans take in more and more acid, through diet, drugs, pollutants, and lifestyle, their bodies have evolved the following measures to keep their blood in relative balance:

1. Hold excess fat in which to store acid.
2. Line arterial walls with fat to prevent collapse.
3. Leech calcium and magnesium from bones to neutralize acids.
4. Draw alkaline stores from bone marrow to neutralize acids.

The reason your body stores fat in your arterial walls is to protect your heart. If the walls were to become thin, the lining of your arteries would deteriorate. Ironically the fat is like a buffer, keeping you safe. Unfortunately, when you get too much fat, it hardens and becomes plaque.

A person cannot be acidic and healthy.

You may be thin. But if you lead an acidic lifestyle it won't matter. Eventually, as more acids enter and build up your body, your body will begin to break down, and the ailments that we associate with old age will catch up with you. These ailments include but are not limited to:

Heart Disease
Coronary Artery Disease
Atherosclerosis
Cancer**
Type 2 Diabetes
Alzheimer's*
Parkinson's*
Osteoporosis
Arthritis
Gout
Infertility*
Erectile Dysfunction*

Stage 2: Anti-Inflammatory Stage
(Days 4-6)

While continuing with what you've been doing thus far, you will add a host of anti-inflammatory herbs to your regimen. These additions will increase your metabolism, burn fat, clear mucus, alleviate the conditions that host parasites, kill (or purge) free radicals, cleanse your lymph system, and prepare your digestive systems for Stage Three.

Benefits: In addition to an increase in the benefits described in Stage One, your body will begin to feel lighter; you will experience even more energy. Blockages in your small intestine will be cleared. People with joint pain, headaches, fatigue, insomnia, will likely find there symptoms begin to disappear.

Burning out the baddies with an anti-inflammatory regimen

Quick summary for those who want to skip ahead: *Some foods cause inflammation. Some foods alleviate inflammation. Over the next six days we will continue reducing the foods that cause inflammation, and begin introducing foods that alleviate inflammation. (Feel free to skip to Chapter 3 or read on)*

(Regarding the section below, the term *foods* refers to both foods and beverages)

Inflammation refers to the body's immune response to conditions that occur within its many systems. Although linked with the Acid Alkaline integrity of the foods one consume a, it is more a measure of the *chemical compounds* within the foods themselves than it is their acid alkaline composition. For the sake of simplicity, let us say that there are three classes of foods:

Foods and Chemicals that <u>Cause</u> Inflammation

White Sugar and High Fructose Corn Syrup: Spikes insulin, raises cytokine levels, host's candida, can lead to fatty liver disease, diabetes, and may change cellular integrity. H.F.C.S. may compromise DNA by affecting *Eicosanoids*.
Replace with: Pure Maple Syrup (in moderation), Pure Stevia, Medjool Dates.

Alcohol: Dehydrates the system, taxes the liver and stomach, kills 'good' bacteria, depletes minerals, disrupts digestion, can lead to cirrhosis.
Replace with: Water, Fresh Vegetable Juice, 'Green' Drink.

Soda and Energy Drinks: Raises cytokine levels, feeds candida, can lead to Fatty Liver Disease and Diabetes, wreaks havoc on white blood cells, many brands contain carcinogens such as Brominated Vegetable Oil and Aspartame.
Replace with: Water, Fresh Vegetable Juice, Green Drink, Yerba Matte, Green Tea.

Red Meat: Raises cholesterol, slows digestion, increases parasite risk, and may putrefy in the small intestine. Recently, the World Health Organization classified red meats as a *high cancer risk* food.
Replace with: Beans, Rice, Legumes, Leafy greens, Starches.

Dairy: Depletes minerals, increases the body's level of Insulin Like Growth Factor. Dairy consumption is directly linked to prostate cancer and may increase risk of colon cancer.
Replace with: Non-Sweetened plant milks (Almond, Rice, Soy, Cashew, Coconut Hemp, Flax)

Unbleached White Flours: Damages cells in lining of blood vessels, promotes candida, hinders digestion of certain proteins when combined with them. Most breads containing Unbleached White Flours have insufficient vitamins or trace minerals.
Replace with: Sprouted breads, ancient grains (kamut, spelt, quinoa, teff, amaranth, sorghum, millet.)

Coffee: (In large amounts) kills good bacteria, taxes the adrenal system, and raises cortisol. Some coffee beans may be treated with known toxins such as formaldehyde, hexane, trichloroethylene, chloroform, acetone, and methanol.
Organic coffee, taken in marginal amounts (about 2-4 ounces per day depending on individual) actually has some benefits.
Replace with: Yerba Matte, Green Tea, Black Tea

Herbs that <u>fight</u> Inflammation

Turmeric: The undisputed king of anti-inflammatory herbs. Turmeric has anti-inflammatory and anti fungal properties, its main compound *Curcumin* has been scientifically proven to help relieve everything from arthritis to allergies. Turmeric lowers cholesterol, helps the liver, and may prevent certain types of cancer.
Tip: Buy turmeric in the bulk section of your supermarket.

Cayenne: In addition to *Capsaicin*, Cayenne contains many *carotenoids* and *flavonoids,* two classes of compounds that attach to free radicals and may prevent cancer. Cayenne stimulates the digestive tract and promotes enzyme production. In addition, Cayenne helps the body rid itself of toxins.
Tip: If you dislike spicy foods, you can offset cayenne by adding a dash to a sweet smoothie (bananas, ice-cubes, cinnamon and almond milk is a great one), this will prevent the spice from overwhelming your palate.

Garlic: Garlic contains many inflammation-busting compounds. Three of the most important are: *allicin, alliin,* and ajoene, all are rich in anti-fungal and anti-bacterial properties. Garlic has been proven to reduce blood pressure, lower LDL cholesterol, and purge lactic acid from muscles.
Tip: 1-2 cloves of garlic is a great addition to fresh vegetable juice.

Ginger: One of the best arthritis relievers in the world, ginger contains an antioxidant called Gingerol-6 which helps relieve and prevent osteoarthritis. Ginger also helps aide digestion and kill parasites such as Salmonella and Trichomonoas. Studies show that ginger drastically improves glycated hemoglobin levels in diabetic and pre-diabetic patients.
Tip: Ginger is stellar at relieving motion sickness.

Cinnamon: Cinnamon contains polyphenols, which help prevent oxidative damage caused by free radicals, repairs body tissue, regulates blood sugar, disrupts the stomachs production of Advanced Glycation End Products. There is evidence that cinnamon *may* help patients with Parkinson's by balancing neurotransmitter levels.
Tip: Eat cinnamon with Oats and raisins, or sprinkle some on an apple wedge.

Tart Cherries: Full of anti-oxidants and anthocyanin's which fight obesity, battle gout, aid in post workout muscle repair, help arthritis flare ups, and may reduce stroke risk.
Tip: Tart cherries are best taken in concentrate. They also contain melatonin which is a great natural sleep aide.

Pepper: Peppers contains *Piperine* which is a natural decongestant, and *carminative* which may help prevent malignant tumors from forming. Pepper's main benefits

deal with the digestive system, killing parasites, preventing gas, and easing constipation.
Tip: Consume pepper with turmeric to get maximum punch.

Cloves: Cloves contain antimicrobial compounds galore. These compounds aide digestion, may prevent cancer, boost immunity, keep blood sugars in check, protect the liver, boost the immune system, controls diabetes, and containing anti-mutagenic properties.
Tip: Clove oil is popular for oral health challenges such as toothaches.

Rosemary: Improves digestion, helps inflammation, protects cellular membranes, prevents tumor growth, may improve cognition and memory in older adults.
Tip: by weight, rosemary has more vitamin C than an orange, so if you're feeling a cold coming on, make a tea with fresh rosemary.

Oregano: Often supplemented as oil, oregano has been proven to fight infection, kill parasites, eliminate free radicals, aide in digestion, relieve symptoms of PMS and Menopause, and lower blood triglyceride levels.
Tip: Oregano oil may help soothe the symptoms associated with PMS and menopause.

Ginseng: Boosts immune system, shortens duration of colds, combats fatigue, may help with erectile dysfunction, supports healthy cholesterol levels.
Tip: Ginseng is purported to help men with sexual fatigue.

Stage 3: Probiotic Gut Reset
(Days 7-9)

On Day 7, you will begin to add specific probiotic foods to your diet that will help replenish your lower digestive systems with good bacteria. This in turn will allow your digestive tract to begin healing. Your lower digestive systems will properly break down and absorb nutrients.

Benefits: An easier time losing weight and keeping it off, reduction in bloating, reduction in insulin resistance, clearing parasites, increased benefits for sufferers of Atherosclerosis, Heart Disease, and Crohn's disease.

Replenish your gut with fat burning macrobiotics!

When I first began teaching my clients that bacteria were partly responsible for both their inability to lose weight and many of their ailments, I was often met with quizzical looks and blank stares. I came to realize that our society has been conditioned to the notion that 'bacteria are bad'. I want to clarify this myth once and for all: Not only are most bacteria 'not bad', most bacteria are essential for maintaining life.

Now, because this is a book outlining a change in diet plan, and not a thesis for a 400 level biology class, let us imagine that there are classes of microorganisms:

1. *Good* Microorganisms (Probiotics): These little organisms serve many functions, including: keeping us alive, healing us from a wide array of problems, preventing us from getting sick, and regulating our weight loss. These are the ones we want to be putting into our bodies.
2. *Bad* Microorganisms (Germs): When these little bacteria get in our systems they (can) make us sick. Some of the most devastating diseases known to science are caused by bacteria, yet it is important to note that simply because a person is a carrier for a strain of bacteria, it does not automatically mean that individual will get sick.
3. *Neutral* Microorganisms: Of the trillions of little organisms in our body, these tiny freeloaders are basically just hanging out. Science has yet to find an immediate harm from their existence, yet can also find no benefits.

Probiotic Bacteria that are wonderful us

There are over 160 known strains of beneficial probiotics. The ones listed below are some of the most well researched and well documented. It's more important to familiarize yourself with the foods that these bacteria are found in, than it is the names and benefits of the bacteria.

Lactobacillus Plantarum
Prevents 'bad' germs from flourishing. Creates a healthy barrier in your small intestine which may prevent dangerous bacteria from penetrating the lining, and\or kill it in the intestines before it can enter your blood stream.
Found in: Kim Chee, Sauerkraut and Supplement form.

Lactobacillus Paracasei
When an individual is healthy, Lactobacillus Paracasei boosts the immune system by boosting energy levels. L Paracasei also aids in the digestion of food and may even help with chronic fatigue, acid indigestion, and diarrhea.
Found in: Kim Chee, Sauerkraut, Fermented Vegetables, Kefir, and Supplement form.

Lactobacillus Salivarius
One of the most important gut bacteria for maintaining a healthy weight. L Salivarius resides with the small intestines and fights against a wide array of pathogenic organisms. Helps prevent bloating, and flatulence from people suffering from Irritable Bowel Syndrome.
Found in: Fermented Vegetables and Supplement form.

Lactobacillus Bulgaricus
L Bulgaricus helps neutralize toxins and kills harmful bacteria by starving it of nutrients. L Bulgaricus may also help other symbiotic bacteria to thrive.
Found in: Miso, Soy, Tempeh, and Supplement form

Streptococcus Thermophiles
One of the most heavily studied probiotics, S. Thermophiles regulates digestion, prevents infections, decreases the chance of kidney stones, and increases HDL. This probiotic is one of the most fundamental at preventing gastrointestinal infections.
Found in: Kim Chee, Sauerkraut, fermented vegetables, and supplement form

*In the list above I offer many sources from which to find these probiotics. I omit dairy products because, in my professional opinion, I feel that deriving ones probiotics from dairy is like quenching ones thirst with seawater. In the short term, you may feel that you are experiencing benefits, however, in the long term, the acidosis and inflammation associated with dairy is generally not worth the trade off (especially for an individual hoping to optimize their weight or improve their health) Feel free to do your own research and draw your own conclusions.

Basic Starter Grocery List

Depending on your dietary needs, this list should see you through most of your 9-day Vibrant Energy Cleanse. However, you are *not* required to purchase everything on this list.

Produce

15-25 medium sized lemons
12-15 bananas
5 cucumbers
4 large carrots
3 large Yams or Sweet Potatoes
3 apples and\or pears
2 tomatoes
2 ripe avocados*
1 beet
¼ watermelon
1 head garlic
1 bag spinach and\or 1 bag arugula
1 bunch kale*
1 onion
1-2 cartons of pure coconut water (no added sugar)

General

3 cans (or 1 bag) of garbanzo beans
2 cans (or 1 bag) of black beans
1 tub Plain Quaker Oats
1 bag raisins*
1 bag prunes or apricots (for snacking)
1 Spice Rack cayenne*
1 Spice Rack cinnamon*
1/8 pound turmeric (Buy in Bulk)*
¼ pound unsalted almonds (Buy in Bulk)
¼ pound brown rice and\or quinoa (Buy in Bulk)*
1 container curry powder (for curry based recipes)
1 bottle Braggs Apple Cider Vinegar (Braggs)*
1 bottle Extra Virgin Olive Oil*
1 loaf sprouted bread (Dave's Killer or Ezekiel)
1-2 blocks firm tofu
1 container of Sauerkraut (Wildbrine, Farmhouse Culture, and Kehoe's Kitchen are my three favorites)
1 Jar *Organic* Kim Chee
2-4 Containers Probiotic Coconut or Almond Yogurt
Psyllium Husk Capsules (50)*
1 container 100 pure maple syrup
Black or Green Tea (if you've been drinking coffee)
1 container unsweetened *plant* milk (Hemp, almond, rice, flax, soy, or cashew)

Supplementing with a Green Drink

For the sake of this course, I am defining 'Green Drink' as a supplemental powder that contains at least **5** of the following ingredients: Wheatgrass, Spirulina, Dulse, Barley grass, Chlorella, Broccoli, Oat grass, Kale, Kelp, and/or Dandelion. Green Drinks are formulated to be extremely alkalizing and provide much needed trace minerals, vitamins, and proteins in an easy to digest form. Green drinks can be found at all Health Food Stores. However, they are about 20% cheaper when purchased online.

Three things to consider:
- Many brands offer single serving packets. These packets allow you to get an idea of what the product tastes like. It's important to select a brand that you like the taste of (or that you can at least tolerate), and bear in mind, if you don't like it at first, your tastes will acclimate as you continue drinking it.
- Although not required for the Vibrant Energy Cleanse I recommend a brand that is organic, contains 'sprouted' proteins (such as amaranth, lentils, pumpkin seeds) and that contains probiotics.
- It is my hope and fervent recommendation that you continue consuming a green drink after your 9 Day cleanse has finished.
- My go to brand is *Garden of Life "Perfect Food"*
- A 240g Tub, usually runs around $42.99 and is worth every penny.

Selecting the Right Juicer

Many years ago, when I was suffering from arthritis, weight gain, and general malaise, I purchased a juicer and began juicing daily. Apart from tasting delicious, juicing is addictive. There is something exciting about watching whole cucumbers get transformed into cool green liquid. To this day, I'm still finding new flavor combinations. (My all time favorite recipe is 8 stalks kale, 2 carrots, 1 lemon, 1 beet, 1 cucumber, 1 slice of ginger, and two cloves of garlic, with 1 tablespoon of the pith stirred back into the juice.) I can't begin to emphasize how critical juicing was to my health then, and I how beneficial it still is to this day. I could write a separate book on the benefits of juicing, but I will keep the list short for the sake of brevity.

- Juicing allows us to consume minerals and vitamins from their purest and most natural sources.
- Many foods are not absorbed by the stomach, juicing alleviates that problem.
- Juicing hydrates the body.
- Many of the most beneficial substances we can consume taste awful. The pungent flavor of raw garlic, the bitter bite of uncooked turmeric, and the spicy hot pain brought on by cayenne can all be offset by the right combinations of fruits and vegetables. Without juice, consuming these and other herbs on a daily basis would be pure punishment.

There are many great juicer brands on the market, but I swear by the Jack Lalanne. Not only is Jack Lalanne the original inventor, but I feel that his model is the best. I've watched my friends and clients invest in other models, only to see them break down with continued use. My Juicer has stood the test of time.

I have attached a link. If I were to make a list of the best $100+ investments I have ever made, my trusty juicer would rank at the very top of the list.

The Importance of a Probiotic Supplement

Toward the end of this 9-day cleanse, your stomach, your small intestine, and your digestive system will be primed to absorb probiotics. So for that reason, I strongly recommend taking a probiotic supplement. This way, if you fail to eat enough fermented foods, (or even if you succeed) you'll know that your gut is truly getting the complete nourishment it needs.

I have tried just about every vegetarian brand on the market, and I swear by ECO Pure Health. When I take it at the end of my cleanse, I feel healthier, and 'lighter'. Whichever supplement you select, make sure it has at least 6 strains of probiotic bacteria and has at least 1 billion active cultures.

If you choose a supplement, you should begin taking capsules on day 6, and continue as directed, until the bottle is empty. This will guarantee that you are reaping the full benefits for months to come.

Basic Schedule

Breakfast

16 ounces *Mean Green Juice*(see recipe) or Green Drink
2 Psyllium capsules with juice
Your choice: alkaline breakfast recipe or alkaline snack

Brunch
16 ounces lemon water
Your choice: alkaline snack or dessert

Lunch
16 ounces lemon water or pure coconut water or Green Drink
Your choice: alkaline lunch recipe (I recommend big salads for lunch)

Late Afternoon
16 ounces lemon water
Your choice: alkaline snack or dessert

Dinner
Your choice: alkaline dinner recipe

Day 0
Preparation day

1. Familiarize yourself with the next 9 days.
2. Stock up on groceries.
3. If you drink coffee, try to cut your in-take by at least half.
4. Inform your friends and family of why you are doing this cleanse and ask them to hold you accountable.
5. Clean all sodas, cookies, pastries, chips, etc. out of your cupboards.
6. If your goal is to lose weight: Take a *before* picture and weigh yourself. *Write your weight down. (Do NOT Weigh yourself a second time until day 9)*
7. Mix some *Green Drink* and start drinking it.
8. Print up a calendar and use a highlighter to mark your nine days. Then get ready to start X-ing out each day as you complete it.

There are 3 things you get do to guarantee your success.
1. Really get associated with why you have chosen to do this cleanse. Write a brief letter to yourself outlining your motivations. If possible, delve in to the pain of what has led you to this moment, and then, describe the pleasure you expect to feel. The more you can get associated with your *why* the better your odds of being successful.
2. Give yourself a legitimate reward for completing day 9. It should be something involving an experience or a treat. Examples might be a new camera, a manicure, a massage, a salsa dancing class, or even taking a vacation day from work. Choose something that will *motivate* you. I do *not* recommend a food or alcohol based reward.
3. Ask someone to hold you accountable. Preferably an individual who you see on a regular basis. Spouses, close friends, and immediate family members can be great choices, however, make sure it's someone who will be supportive of your endeavor.

Day 1

It's day one! Follow the itinerary as best you can. I do not recommend doing any strenuous exercise today.

1. Hydration is vital. Drink <u>lots</u> of lemon water, Green Drink and fresh, homemade vegetable juice. I recommend keeping a 1-gallon jug of purified water and drinking it throughout the day. It is crucial to drink water before you feel thirsty and before you eat.
2. Remember to plan ahead, bring salads to work, have alkaline snacks (apricots, prunes, almond and raisin blend, apple wedges, blueberries, bananas etc.) preplanned and ready to go, and remember, if you are hungry, EAT SOMETHING!
3. It's okay if you don't like the flavor of some new foods yet. Over time your palate will acclimate.
4. If you get a headache today, it is likely either due to sugar withdrawal or caffeine withdrawal. You can taper sugar withdrawal by eating some Medjool dates, and consuming 1 tsp. of pure maple syrup (do not consume more than 2 tsp. per day). Caffeine headaches can be banished by drinking some yerba matte tea. If you are typically a coffee drinker, feel free to drink 2 ounces of black coffee. Do not consume more than 4 ounces. The headaches <u>will</u> pass. Although some dieticians and health experts oppose ibuprofen and/or aspirin, I take them during this period, if concerned, ask a doctor.
5. It is important to chew your food. Chewing has many benefits, including breaking down foods so they can be properly absorbed. This in turn reduces hunger. If you are consuming cooked foods, get in the habit of chewing each bite 30 times.

Day 2

As the acids leave your body, you may begin to experience headaches, back aches, and joint pain. This is a sign that your body is acidic, and that you should keep going. Your body is using this opportunity to rid itself of toxins.

1. Hydrate! Hydrate! Hydrate! Your pee should be as clear as water today, all day!
2. When making your juice, you may wish to add a scoop of the pith (pith is the fibrous material left over in the juice bucket) this will add more fiber to your diet, which in turn will help you eliminate.
3. Juicer tip: Weather permitting, take the non-electrical parts of your juicer outside and blast away the pith with a garden hose, you'll find this much easier than cleaning the parts in the sink.
4. Sliced apple wedges with smears of avocado will be a great, alkalizing snack today.
5. If you feel a bit cranky today, go for a walk and take some deep breaths.
6. If you feel unbearable sugar cravings, add 2 tsp. of maple syrup to your lemon water.
7. Remember to take your Psyllium supplement.

Day 3

Today will likely be another day of detoxification. Your body will continue flushing the acids out of your system, dislodging the food residues that may be residing in your small intestine, and resolving its issue with candida and sugar addiction.

1. This may sound redundant but the most import thing you can do is to continually hydrate with lemon water, green drink, and fresh vegetable juice. If you feel unbearable sugar cravings, add 2 tsp. of maple syrup to your lemon water.
2. A bag of raisins and almonds mixed together is a nice, nourishing snack.
3. If you live in or near a large city you may wish to try a Raw Food Vegan Restaurant. Most cities have them, and pretty much everything on the menu is super alkalizing and contains anti-inflammatory ingredients. Invite a friend with this line: *When was the last time you tried something totally different and exciting?*
4. If you have access to a sauna or a hot tub, today would be a great day to use it. Use best judgment.
5. My hope is that, after today, you will have consumed at least 3 leafy green salads. If you haven't had a salad yet, make a spinach salad with some apple slices, raisins, avocado, tomato, and a dash of Extra Virgin Olive Oil and Apple Cider Vinegar.
6. Nutritional Yeast is a wonderful product high in B-12 and other hard to find vitamins.
7. I'm willing to bet that you've had periods of high energy and periods of crankiness, and possibly headaches and foggy thinking. After today it gets both easier and more fun.

PHASE II

Day 4

Congratulations on making it to Phase II! Over the next three days you will continue with what you've been doing thus far. Follow the outlined meal plan and make sure you keep drinking lots of green drink, lemon water, and fresh vegetable juice. The added anti-inflammatory herbs that we introduce may not seem like much of a change, but the positive effects they have on your immune system, digestive system, and your blood will be anything but meager!

Twice a day:
Add 1 tsp. turmeric powder and ¼ tsp. cayenne pepper to your fresh vegetable juice or green drink. If you do this and nothing else for Phase II you will feel noticeably better.

Once a day:
Add 1-2 raw peeled garlic cloves to your fresh vegetable juice. You may increase your carrots or apples to offset pungency.

Once a day:
Ginger: You may already be using Ginger, but if you haven't been add a piece about the size of a human thumb to your juice.

Cinnamon: Sneak in Cinnamon wherever you can.

Day 5

After today you should start to feel noticeably better. Your skin will start to glow, you may feel like your thoughts are 'clearer' and that your concentration is better. If you suffer from day to day aches and pains you will start noticing a marked improvement.

1. Anti-Inflammatory herbs are most effective when taken on an empty or half empty stomach. This is why I recommend adding them to your juice or lemon water when you first wake up in the morning.
2. Add Rosemary, Basil, Sage, Black Pepper, Clove, Oregano, and Licorice to anything and everything.
3. If you have access to tart cherries, fresh cranberries, or pomegranate seeds, buy some and nibble on them, they are three of the greatest anti-inflammatory foods.
4. Consuming Black pepper and Turmeric together magnifies the properties of both.
5. Many women enjoy the benefits of Oregano oil, while men may see more benefits from Saw Palmetto.
6. I do not recommend take Turmeric or Cayenne two hours before bed, as these herbs may make it harder to fall asleep. On the other hand, I strongly recommend taking lavender and tart cherry concentrate at this time, as they make it easier to fall asleep.

Day 6

Take a look in the mirror and see how your skin is looking. Take a deep breath and feel if you don't breathe a little easier. If you are used to feeling tired and run down, pause for a few moments and see if you don't feel a bit 'lighter'. Over the next few days, these feelings will magnify exponentially.

1. Green tea is full of anti-inflammatory properties, and it provides a nice, but nominal caffeine buzz.
2. Today, add a bit more turmeric and a dash more cayenne to your juice.
3. Drink lots and lots of fresh water today!
4. Have you tried any of the desserts yet?
5. Tonight, review the next chapter and make sure you are stocked up on probiotic, gut healing foods (Kombucha, Kefir, Miso, Tempeh, Natto, Yogurt, Sauerkraut, Kim Chee, and Fermented foods)

Phase III

Day 7

Congratulations on making it to Phase III. For the next three days we will continue phases 1 and 2 while stacking a new phase: adding gut healing, probiotics to your regimen. These probiotics will improve your digestion, lessen your hunger, and help increase your metabolism.

Continue Phases I and II as normal but add:

Three times per day
1. Add 1 Tsp. Apple Cider Vinegar to your lemon water three times per day.

Once per day:

1. Consume one 12 ounce serving of Kombucha.
2. Consumer at least one cup of Raw Organic Kim Chee or Raw Organic Sauerkraut.
3. Consume one serving of miso soup or 1 serving of tempeh per day.
4. If available, consume Kefir products, Tempeh, or Natto, (Asian Supermarkets)
5. I strongly recommend a pro-biotic supplement.

Day 8

Today is the second to last day! Today would be a great day to try experimenting! Add some Sauerkraut to a spinach salad or add some Kim Chee to some rice. Get your probiotics anyway you can!

1. There are many different types of Kombucha, experiment with different brands and different flavors.
2. A little maple syrup in your apple cider vinegar will make it taste pleasant.
3. Many people ferment their own foods in jars and make their own Kombucha. Both are easy and fun, if you are the crafty type, you may wish to do some research.
4. Most labels will say if fermented foods contain probiotic cultures. Don't be afraid to do some research on the Internet.
5. Get ready for your last day!

Day 9

The finish line is in site! Don't give up now. Really try to go all out today, by now you know how to do it, so finish in style!

1. Follow through with Day 9 until the end of the day to reap the full benefits of the cleanse.
2. Make sure you use up the last of your 9 day old produce (and hopefully buy more!)
3. Tonight, make a log of how you are feeling. Does your 'mood' or 'energy' feel lighter?
4. Take a picture of yourself. Does your skin look clearer?

Congratulations

You deserve an enormous congratulations! Your body has achieved acid alkaline integrity, your immune system has been rebooted, and your gut is flourishing with healthy bacteria.

1. If your goal was to lose weight than weigh yourself.
2. Celebrate with a spa day, or a massage.
3. Try to appreciate how you are feeling. Really get in tune with how things feel.
4. Send me an Email at alkalineintegrity@gmail.com tell us how you are doing. What did you like, what didn't you like?
5. Can you think of any friends who would benefit from this cleanse?

Continuing on

Now, I would like to challenge you to do the following for 7 more days.

1. Continue drinking at least 1 quart of lemon water per day.
2. Continue eating one large leafy green salad every 2 days.
3. Continue with your supplements.
5. Refrain from dairy products, red meat, soda, energy drinks, and blended coffee drinks.
6. Continue taking turmeric and cayenne.
7. Continue Juicing and drinking green drink.

That's all!

www.ingramcontent.com/pod-product-compliance
Lightning Source LLC
Chambersburg PA
CBHW050837290526
45792CB00001B/426